REAL FOOD FOR PREGNANCY

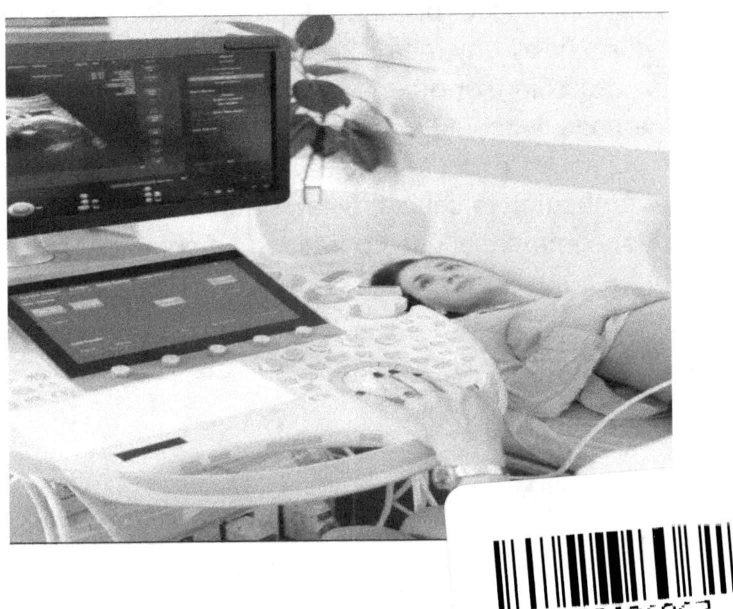

"Nutrient-Rich Eating for a Healthy
Pregnancy Journey"

EMMA LYNCH

TABLE OF CONTENTS

INTRODUCTION

Pregnancy is a remarkable and transformative journey in a woman's life, filled with anticipation, wonder, and a deep desire for the well-being of both mother and child. It's a time when the body undergoes incredible changes, and proper nutrition becomes paramount. In this book, "Real Food for Pregnancy," we will embark on a journey of discovering the nutritional wisdom that can empower expectant mothers to make the best choices for both their own and their developing child's health.

Pregnancy nutrition goes far beyond simply satisfying hunger; it's about providing your body with the essential nutrients required for optimal growth and development. The real food approach emphasizes the importance of wholesome, unprocessed, and nutrient-dense foods as the foundation for a healthy pregnancy. It's about making informed choices and enjoying a variety of delicious, nourishing foods that can support your well-being and enhance your pregnancy experience.

Throughout this book, we will delve into the fundamentals of nutrition during pregnancy, explore the benefits of incorporating real food into your diet, and provide practical guidance, meal planning tips, and a collection of delicious recipes that will make the journey to a healthy pregnancy a fulfilling and satisfying one. Whether you're a first-time mom or have experienced pregnancy before, this book aims to empower you with the knowledge and tools to make real food a central part of your pregnancy, helping you create a nourishing environment for both you and your baby.

So, let's begin this transformative journey of discovery and empowerment, and explore the world of "Real Food for Pregnancy.".

THE IMPORTANCE OF NUTRITION DURING PREGNANCY

Nutrition during pregnancy is a critical factor in ensuring the health and well-being of both the mother and the developing baby. It plays a pivotal role in supporting the various stages of pregnancy, from conception to postpartum, and has a lasting impact on the child's long-term health. Here are some key reasons highlighting the importance of nutrition during pregnancy:

1. **Fetal Development:** Proper nutrition provides essential building blocks for the development of the

baby. Adequate intake of nutrients, such as folic acid, iron, calcium, and various vitamins, is necessary for the formation of the baby's organs, bones, and brain.

2. **Maternal Health:** Pregnancy places increased demands on the mother's body. Nutrient-rich foods help support the physiological changes, maintain healthy body weight, and reduce the risk of pregnancy complications like gestational diabetes and pre-eclampsia.

3. **Immune System Support:** A well-balanced diet boosts the immune system, helping the mother's body defend against infections and illnesses, which is especially important during pregnancy when the immune system may be somewhat compromised.

4. **Energy Levels:** Pregnancy often leads to increased fatigue. Proper nutrition provides the necessary energy to combat this fatigue and helps the mother stay active and engaged in daily life.

5. **Blood Volume and Circulation:** Nutrients like iron are crucial for the production of red blood cells and maintaining proper blood circulation. This helps prevent anemia, which is common in pregnancy.

6. **Brain and Cognitive Development:** Omega-3 fatty acids, found in foods like fish and nuts, are essential for the development of the baby's brain

and nervous system. They also support the mother's mental well-being.

7. **Growth and Weight Gain:** Appropriate weight gain during pregnancy is vital, and a balanced diet contributes to healthy growth. It reduces the risk of low birth weight and associated health problems.

8. **Postpartum Recovery:** Good nutrition during pregnancy also sets the stage for a smoother postpartum period. It aids in healing, breastfeeding, and overall recovery.

9. **Long-Term Health:** The nutritional choices made during pregnancy can influence the child's health later in life. A well-nourished mother is more likely to have a healthy baby who is at lower risk of chronic health issues like obesity and diabetes.

10. **Nutritional Quality Over Quantity:** It's not just about eating more; it's about eating the right foods. Real, whole foods provide a wide range of nutrients, whereas processed and fast foods are often empty in terms of nutrition.

In essence, nutrition during pregnancy is a cornerstone of a healthy, successful pregnancy. It's about making informed choices, embracing a balanced diet, and ensuring that both mother and baby receive the nourishment they need to thrive.

CHAPTER ONE

UNDERSTANDING YOUR NUTRITIONAL NEEDS

Pregnancy is a unique and transformative period in a woman's life, and it comes with increased nutritional requirements to support both the mother's health and the development of the baby. Understanding your nutritional needs during pregnancy is crucial for ensuring a healthy and successful journey. Here are some critical considerations:

1. **Macronutrients:**
   - *Carbohydrates:* Carbohydrates provide energy and are important for maintaining blood glucose levels. Fruits, vegetables, and whole grains are great sources of complex carbs.
   - *Proteins:* Proteins are essential for the growth and development of the baby. Lean meats, poultry, fish, beans, and dairy products are good protein sources.
   - *Fats:* Healthy fats, especially omega-3 fatty acids, support the development of the baby's brain and nervous system. Sources include fatty fish, avocados, and nuts.

2. **Micronutrients:**

   - *Folate (Folic Acid):* Folate is crucial for preventing birth defects. It's found in leafy greens, legumes, and fortified cereals.
   - *Iron:* Iron is necessary for preventing anemia and supporting the increased blood volume during pregnancy. Red meat, poultry, and beans are iron-rich foods.
   - *Calcium:* The development of the baby's bones depends on calcium. Leafy greens, plant-based milks with added nutrients, and dairy products are excellent sources.
   - *Vitamins:* Vitamins like vitamin D, vitamin C, and vitamin A play essential roles in maintaining the health of both mother and baby. Ensure a variety of fruits and vegetables in your diet.
   - *Minerals:* Minerals like magnesium and zinc are required for various bodily functions and should be obtained through a balanced diet.

3. **Hydration:**
   - Staying well-hydrated is crucial during pregnancy. Adequate water intake helps with digestion, circulation, and the amniotic fluid that surrounds the baby.

4. **Caloric Intake:**
   - While the emphasis is on nutrient-dense foods, you'll also need some additional calories during pregnancy, particularly in the second and third trimesters. However, this doesn't mean eating for two; it means making your calories count by choosing nutritious foods.

5. **Supplements:**
   - In some cases, healthcare providers may recommend prenatal supplements to ensure that you're meeting your nutritional needs, especially for folic acid and iron.

6. **Gestational Changes:**
   - Nutritional needs can vary throughout pregnancy, so it's essential to adapt your diet as your body and the baby's requirements change.

7. **Consulting with a Healthcare Provider:**
   - It's crucial to work with your healthcare provider to determine your specific nutritional needs, especially if you have underlying health conditions or are at risk for complications.

Understanding and meeting your nutritional needs during pregnancy is vital for a healthy and successful pregnancy journey. Every woman's needs can vary, so seeking guidance from healthcare professionals and adopting a real food approach to nutrition can help ensure that you and your baby receive the essential nutrients for a thriving and fulfilling pregnancy.

MACRONUTRIENTS

Macronutrients in Pregnancy

During pregnancy, macronutrients—carbohydrates, proteins, and fats—are essential components of your diet that provide the energy and building blocks needed for both you and your developing baby. Understanding how to balance these macronutrients is crucial for a healthy pregnancy:

1. **Carbohydrates:**
   - **Role:** The body uses carbs as its main energy source. They provide glucose for your cells and help maintain blood glucose levels.
   - **Pregnancy Importance:** During pregnancy, carbohydrates are essential for providing energy to support the growing demands of your body and the developing baby.
   - **Sources:** Opt for complex carbohydrates found in whole grains (brown rice, whole wheat, quinoa), fruits, vegetables, and legumes. These are high in fiber, which helps with digestion, and they offer lasting energy.

2. **Proteins:**
   - **Role:** Proteins are the building blocks of the body. They are crucial for the development of your baby's tissues, including muscles, organs, and the placenta.
   - **Pregnancy Importance:** Protein needs increase during pregnancy to support the growth of the baby and the expansion of maternal blood volume.
   - **Sources:** Lean sources of protein include poultry, fish, lean meats, eggs, dairy products,

legumes, and tofu. These provide essential amino acids needed for both you and your baby.

3. **Fats:**
   - **Role:** Fats serve multiple functions, including energy storage, protecting organs, and aiding in the absorption of fat-soluble vitamins.
   - **Pregnancy Importance:** Healthy fats are important during pregnancy for the development of the baby's brain and nervous system.
   - **Sources:** Include sources of healthy fats in your diet, such as avocados, nuts, seeds, olive oil, and fatty fish like salmon. Omega-3 fatty acids, particularly DHA, are crucial for the baby's brain and eye development.

It's important to note that while macronutrients are critical, the quality of the foods you choose matters. Opt for nutrient-dense sources of carbohydrates, proteins, and fats. Whole, unprocessed foods should be the foundation of your diet during pregnancy, as they provide a wide array of vitamins, minerals, and other essential nutrients.

Additionally, the balance of macronutrients in your diet should reflect your specific needs, which may vary depending on your activity level, pre-pregnancy weight, and any existing health conditions. Consulting with a healthcare provider or a registered dietitian can help you create a personalized nutrition plan to meet your unique macronutrient requirements during pregnancy.

MICRONUTRIENTS

Micronutrients are essential vitamins and minerals that your body needs in smaller quantities compared to macronutrients but are no less important during pregnancy. These micronutrients play a vital role in supporting the health of both the expectant mother and the developing baby. Here are some of the key micronutrients and their importance during pregnancy:

1. **Folate (Folic Acid):**
   - **Importance:** Folate is crucial for preventing neural tube defects in the baby. It is also required for the production of DNA and the development of cells.
   - **Sources:** Leafy greens, fortified cereals, legumes, and supplements (often recommended in pregnancy).

2. **Iron:**
   - **Importance:** Iron is necessary for preventing anemia and for the production of hemoglobin, which carries oxygen in the blood.
   - **Sources:** Red meat, poultry, fish, beans, lentils, and iron-fortified foods.

3. **Calcium:**

   - **Importance:** Calcium supports the baby's bone and teeth development and helps maintain the mother's bone health.
   - **Sources:** Dairy products, fortified plant-based milks, leafy greens, and almonds.

4. **Vitamin D:**
   - **Importance:** Vitamin D is essential for calcium absorption and bone health in both the mother and baby.
   - **Sources:** Sunlight exposure, fatty fish, and vitamin D-fortified foods. Supplements may be recommended if vitamin D levels are insufficient.

5. **Vitamin C:**
   - **Importance:** Vitamin C supports the body's immune system and aids in the absorption of iron from plant-based sources.
   - **Sources:** Citrus fruits, strawberries, bell peppers, and broccoli are all good choices.

6. **Vitamin A:**
   - **Importance:** Vitamin A is necessary for the baby's eye and skin development and helps with immune function.
   - **Sources:** Liver, sweet potatoes, carrots, and spinach (in moderation).

7. **Vitamin E:**
   - **Importance:** Vitamin E is an antioxidant that helps protect cells from damage.
   - **Sources:** Nuts, seeds, and spinach.

8. **B Vitamins (B6, B12, Niacin, Riboflavin, Thiamin):**
   - **Importance:** These B vitamins are involved in various processes, including metabolism and energy production.
   - **Sources:** Meat, fish, poultry, dairy products, and whole grains.

9. **Minerals (Magnesium, Zinc):**
   - **Importance:** These minerals support various bodily functions, including muscle and nerve function, immune health, and wound healing.
   - **Sources:** Nuts, whole grains, lean meats, and seafood.

It's important to note that a well-balanced and varied diet that includes a wide range of whole, unprocessed foods is the best way to ensure you're getting these essential micronutrients. However, some pregnant women may require supplements, such as prenatal vitamins, to meet their nutritional needs adequately. Consulting with a healthcare provider or a registered dietitian can help you determine if supplementation is necessary and ensure that you are meeting your specific micronutrient requirements during pregnancy.

SPECIAL CONSIDERATIONS

Pregnancy can present unique dietary challenges, especially for women with specific health conditions or dietary preferences. Here are some special conditions and considerations during pregnancy:

1. **Vegetarian and Vegan Pregnancy:**
   - *Challenges:* Vegetarian and vegan diets can be nutritionally adequate during pregnancy, but careful planning is necessary to ensure you get essential nutrients like protein, iron, calcium, vitamin B12, and omega-3 fatty acids.
   - *Solutions:* Incorporate a variety of plant-based protein sources (legumes, tofu, tempeh), fortified foods (for B12), calcium-rich foods (fortified plant-based milks, leafy greens), and consider omega-3 supplements derived from algae.

2. **Food Allergies and Sensitivities:**
   - *Challenges:* If you have food allergies or sensitivities, it's essential to avoid your allergens. This can sometimes limit food choices.
   - *Solutions:* Work with a healthcare provider or dietitian to create a safe and balanced meal plan, ensuring you still get all the necessary nutrients while avoiding allergenic foods.

3. **Gestational Diabetes:**
   - *Challenges:* Gestational diabetes can affect blood sugar levels during pregnancy, necessitating dietary adjustments to control glucose.
   - *Solutions:* Focus on complex carbohydrates, monitor blood sugar levels, and limit sugary foods and refined carbs. Consult with a healthcare provider for a personalized plan.

4. **Celiac Disease:**
   - *Challenges:* Celiac disease requires strict avoidance of gluten-containing foods, which can make it challenging to get enough fiber and certain nutrients.
   - *Solutions:* Seek gluten-free whole grains, such as quinoa, rice, and gluten-free oats, and ensure that you're consuming a variety of nutrient-dense, naturally gluten-free foods.

5. **Vegetarian and Vegan Pregnancy:**
   - *Challenges:* Vegetarian and vegan diets can be nutritionally adequate during pregnancy, but careful planning is necessary to ensure you get essential nutrients like protein, iron, calcium, vitamin B12, and omega-3 fatty acids.
   - *Solutions:* Incorporate a variety of plant-based protein sources (legumes, tofu, tempeh), fortified foods (for B12), calcium-rich foods (fortified plant-based milks, leafy greens), and consider omega-3 supplements derived from algae.

6. **Lactose Intolerance:**
   - *Challenges:* If you're lactose intolerant, you may need alternative sources of calcium and vitamin D.
   - *Solutions:* Choose lactose-free dairy products or lactase supplements, and consider fortified plant-based milks or other calcium-rich foods.

7. **Multiple Pregnancies (Twins, Triplets):**

   - *Challenges:* Carrying multiple babies can increase nutritional needs.
   - *Solutions:* Work closely with a healthcare provider to monitor your nutritional requirements, which may include additional calories, protein, and certain nutrients.

8. **Underweight or Overweight:**
   - *Challenges:* Being significantly underweight or overweight can affect the baby's health and require specific dietary considerations.
   - *Solutions:* Consult with a healthcare provider or dietitian to create a tailored nutrition plan to address weight-related concerns and optimize the health of you and your baby.

It's important to remember that every pregnancy is unique, and these special conditions should be managed on an individual basis. Seeking guidance from a healthcare provider or a registered dietitian can help ensure that you address these specific needs and maintain a healthy and balanced diet during pregnancy.

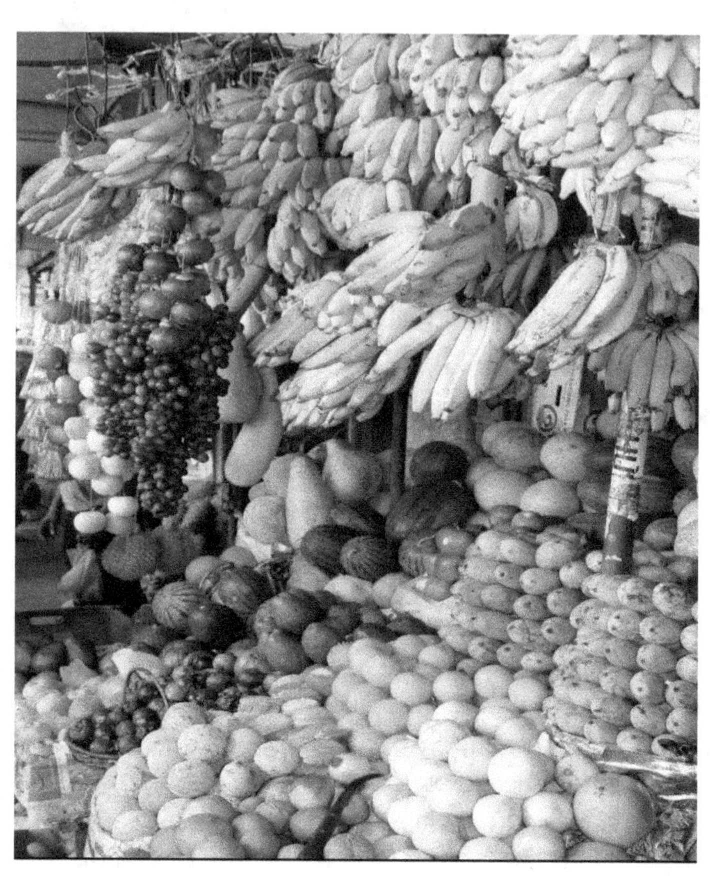

CHAPTER TWO

BUILDING A REAL FOOD FOUNDATION

Creating a real food foundation for pregnancy means prioritizing whole, unprocessed, and nutrient-dense foods to support the health of both the mother and the developing baby. Here are key steps to build this foundation:

1. **Choose Whole Foods:**
   - Choose items that are as near to their original state as you can. Fresh fruits and vegetables, whole grains, lean proteins, and unprocessed dairy products should form the basis of your diet.

2. **Prioritize Organic When Possible:**
   - Eating organic food can lessen your exposure to toxins and pesticides. While it's not always necessary, consider choosing organic options, especially for items known to have higher pesticide residues.

3. **Food Safety:**
   - Be vigilant about food safety during pregnancy to reduce the risk of foodborne illnesses. This includes proper food storage, cooking temperatures, and avoiding raw or undercooked seafood, eggs, and meats.

4. **Balanced Meals:**
   - Create balanced meals that include a variety of macronutrients (carbohydrates, proteins, fats) to provide sustained energy. Incorporate a rainbow of fruits and vegetables to ensure a range of vitamins and minerals.

5. **Fiber-Rich Foods:**
   - Foods high in fiber, such as whole grains, legumes, and fruits, support healthy digestion and help prevent constipation, a common issue during pregnancy.

6. **Healthy Fats:**
   - Incorporate foods like avocados, nuts, seeds, and fatty fish into your diet as sources of healthy fats. Omega-3 fatty acids, in particular, are vital for brain development.

7. **Lean Proteins:**
   - Choose lean sources of protein, like poultry, fish, beans, and legumes. Protein is necessary for the growth and development of the infant.

8. **Adequate Hydration:**
   - To stay well hydrated, sip lots of water. Urinary tract infections are among the problems that can arise from dehydration.

9. **Limit Processed Foods:**

- Minimize the consumption of highly processed and sugary foods, as they often lack essential nutrients and can lead to excessive weight gain and blood sugar fluctuations.

10. **Supplements:**
   - If recommended by your healthcare provider, take prenatal supplements to fill in any nutritional gaps. Prenatal vitamins often provide additional folic acid, iron, and other essential nutrients.

11. **Mindful Eating:**
   - Practice mindful eating, paying attention to hunger and fullness cues, and savoring the flavors and textures of real, whole foods.

12. **Variety Is Key:**
   - Ensure a variety of foods in your diet to receive a broad spectrum of nutrients. Different foods offer different nutritional benefits.

13. **Consult a Healthcare Provider or Dietitian:**
   - Work with a healthcare provider or a registered dietitian to create a personalized nutrition plan that addresses your specific needs and concerns during pregnancy.

Building a real food foundation during pregnancy is about making informed and conscious choices to provide the essential nutrients required for a healthy pregnancy. It's a journey of embracing wholesome, nourishing foods that support the well-being of both you and your growing baby.

CHOOSING WHOLE FOOD

Choosing Whole Foods for a Healthy Pregnancy

Selecting whole foods during pregnancy is a fundamental part of building a nutritious and balanced diet. Whole foods are minimally processed or refined, and they offer a wealth of essential nutrients. Here's how to choose and incorporate whole foods into your pregnancy diet:

1. **Fruits and Vegetables:**
   - Opt for fresh, seasonal fruits and vegetables whenever possible. Minerals, vitamins, and antioxidants abound in them. Aim to include a variety of colors to ensure you get a wide range of nutrients.
   - Consider buying organic produce, especially for items like berries and leafy greens, which tend to have higher pesticide residues.

2. **Whole Grains:**
   - Opt for whole grains such as whole-grain pasta, brown rice, quinoa, oats, and whole wheat. These grains provide complex carbohydrates, fiber, and various nutrients.

   - Avoid refined grains like white rice and white bread, as they lack the fiber and nutrients found in whole grains.

3. **Lean Proteins:**
   - Prioritize lean sources of protein, such as skinless poultry, fish, beans, lentils, tofu, and low-fat dairy products. These options offer essential amino acids without excessive saturated fat.
   - Limit processed and red meats, which can be high in saturated fats and sodium.

4. **Healthy Fats:**
   - Include foods high in avocados, nuts, seeds, and olive oil in your diet as sources of healthy fats. These fats provide monounsaturated and polyunsaturated fats that support overall health.
   - Incorporate fatty fish like salmon, which is rich in omega-3 fatty acids, important for the baby's brain and nervous system development.

5. **Dairy and Dairy Alternatives:**
   - If you consume dairy, choose plain, unsweetened, and low-fat or reduced-fat options. Dairy products offer calcium and protein.
   - For those with lactose intolerance or following a vegan diet, consider fortified plant-based milks (e.g., almond milk, soy milk) to ensure calcium intake.

6. **Legumes:**

- Legumes, such as beans, lentils, and chickpeas, are a great source of fiber and plant-based protein. They're also rich in various vitamins and minerals.
  - Incorporate legumes into soups, salads, and main dishes to boost your nutrient intake.

7. **Nuts and Seeds:**
   - Snack on unsalted nuts and seeds, which provide healthy fats, protein, and a variety of vitamins and minerals. Nuts like flaxseeds, chia seeds, walnuts, and almonds are good choices.

8. **Spices and Herbs:**
   - Flavor your meals with herbs and spices like basil, oregano, turmeric, and cinnamon. These can enhance the taste of your dishes without adding extra sodium or sugar.

9. **Minimize Processed Foods:**
   - Reduce your consumption of processed and packaged foods, as they often contain added sugars, unhealthy fats, and excessive sodium. These can lead to weight gain and blood sugar fluctuations.

10. **Read Labels:**
    - When buying packaged foods, read ingredient labels and choose products with minimal additives, preservatives, and artificial ingredients.

Choosing whole foods during pregnancy helps ensure you're getting the most nutrition from your diet. Whole foods provide essential nutrients that support your health and the development of your baby. A balanced and mindful approach to your food choices will contribute to a healthy and fulfilling pregnancy.

ORGANIC VS CONVENTIONAL

The choice between organic and conventional foods during pregnancy is a common consideration. Both have their advantages and potential drawbacks. To assist you decide, consider the following comparison:

Organic Foods:

1. **Reduced Pesticide Exposure:**
   - Organic foods are grown without synthetic pesticides or herbicides. This can be particularly appealing during pregnancy to minimize exposure to potentially harmful chemicals.

2. **No Genetically Modified Organisms (GMOs):**
   - Organic regulations prohibit the use of genetically modified organisms (GMOs). This may be important to some individuals who prefer non-GMO foods.

3. **Environmental Impact:**

- Organic farming practices often prioritize sustainability and reduce the environmental impact of agriculture.

Conventional Foods:

1. **Cost-Effective:**
   - Conventional foods are typically more affordable than organic options, making them a practical choice for many families.

2. **Availability and Variety:**
   - Conventional foods are more widely available and offer a broader range of choices in terms of products and brands.

3. **Nutritional Content:**
   - Nutrient content can be similar between organic and conventional foods. The most important factor is overall diet quality and variety.

Considerations for Pregnancy:

1. **Pesticide Exposure:** If you're concerned about pesticide exposure, especially for fruits and vegetables with higher pesticide residues, you may opt for organic options when available. Washing produce thoroughly can also help reduce pesticide residues.

2. **Budget:** If budget constraints are a consideration, you can prioritize organic choices for

foods that tend to have higher pesticide residues (often referred to as the "Dirty Dozen") and opt for conventional for others.

3. **Balanced Diet:** Regardless of whether you choose organic or conventional, focusing on a balanced diet rich in whole, unprocessed foods is essential. A range of fruits, vegetables, lean proteins, and whole grains should all be a part of your diet.

4. **Local and Seasonal Foods:** Whenever possible, consider buying local and seasonal produce. These items are often fresher and may be grown with fewer pesticides, whether they are certified organic or not.

5. **Food Safety:** Ensure that you follow proper food safety practices regardless of the type of food you choose. This includes washing fruits and vegetables, cooking meat thoroughly, and handling food with clean hands and utensils.

Ultimately, the decision between organic and conventional foods during pregnancy is a personal one. It may depend on your budget, values, and specific concerns. Whether you choose organic or conventional, maintaining a well-balanced and nutritious diet is the most important factor for a healthy pregnancy. You can also discuss your dietary choices with your healthcare provider to address any specific concerns you may have.

FOOD SAFETY DURING PREGNANCY

Food safety is of paramount importance during pregnancy to protect both the expectant mother and the developing baby from the risk of foodborne illnesses. Hormonal changes during pregnancy can weaken the immune system, making pregnant women more susceptible to certain infections. Here are essential guidelines to ensure food safety during pregnancy:

1. **Wash Hands Thoroughly:**
   - Always wash your hands with warm, soapy water before handling or preparing food. This helps prevent the transfer of harmful bacteria to food.

2. **Clean and Sanitize Cooking Surfaces:**
   - Keep kitchen countertops, cutting boards, and utensils clean and sanitized to avoid cross-contamination. Use different chopping boards for produce and uncooked meats.

3. **Rinse Fruits and Vegetables:**
   - Thoroughly rinse fresh fruits and vegetables under running water to remove dirt and potential contaminants. Use a brush for produce with thicker skins.

4. **Avoid Raw or Undercooked Meat and Seafood:**

- Cook all meat and seafood to safe internal temperatures to kill harmful bacteria. Avoid undercooked or raw meats, including sushi, and unpasteurized seafood.

5. **Limit Processed and Deli Meats:**
   - Processed and deli meats may carry the risk of listeria contamination. If you choose to consume these meats, heat them to a safe temperature to kill potential bacteria.

6. **Pasteurized Dairy Products:**
   - Consume only pasteurized dairy products to avoid the risk of harmful bacteria. Check labels to ensure that products are pasteurized.

7. **Avoid Soft Cheeses and Unpasteurized Dairy:**
   - Soft cheeses like feta, brie, and queso fresco, as well as unpasteurized dairy products, can carry the risk of listeria. Opt for hard cheeses or heat soft cheeses until they're steaming hot before consumption.

8. **Safe Egg Handling:**
   - Cook eggs thoroughly until the yolks and whites are firm to avoid the risk of salmonella. Avoid foods that contain raw or undercooked eggs, such as homemade mayonnaise or raw cookie dough.

9. **Be Cautious with Fresh Sprouts:**

- Fresh sprouts, like alfalfa and mung bean sprouts, can harbor harmful bacteria. Cook or avoid them during pregnancy.

10. **Food Storage:**
   - Refrigerate perishable foods promptly to keep them fresh and safe to eat. Follow recommended storage times for leftovers and ensure your refrigerator is set at or below 40°F (4°C).

11. **Be Mindful of Mercury in Fish:**
   - High levels of mercury in some fish can be hazardous to the developing baby's nervous system. Avoid or limit consumption of high-mercury fish like shark, swordfish, king mackerel, and tilefish. Instead, choose fish lower in mercury, such as salmon, trout, and sardines.

12. **Stay Informed:**
   - Stay up to date on food recalls and advisories. The Food and Drug Administration (FDA) and the Centers for Disease Control and Prevention (CDC) provide information on food safety alerts.

13. **Eating Out:**
   - When dining out, be cautious about the source and handling of your food. Ensure that meat and seafood are thoroughly cooked, and ask about the safety of salads and unpasteurized dairy products.

Food safety during pregnancy is essential to protect the health of both you and your baby. Following these guidelines and being mindful of what you eat can help reduce the risk of foodborne illnesses and ensure a safe and healthy pregnancy. If you have specific concerns or questions about food safety, consult with your healthcare provider or a registered dietitian.

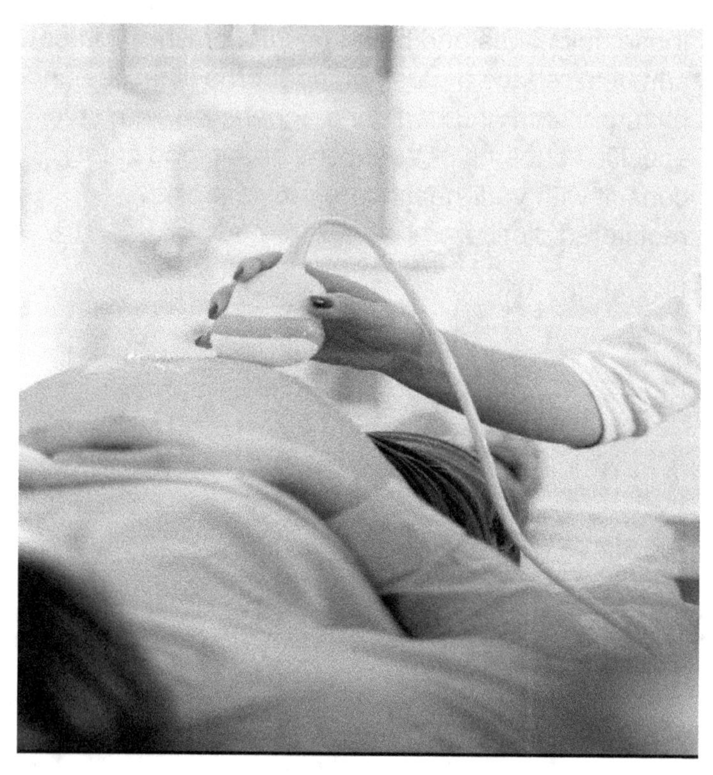

CHAPTER THREE

MEAL PLANNING AND RECIPES

Meal planning during pregnancy is an essential part of ensuring you get the right nutrients to support your health and the development of your baby. Here's a step-by-step guide to help you plan meals and some recipe ideas to get you started:

Step 1: Set Your Nutritional Goals

Before planning your meals, consider your specific nutritional needs during pregnancy. Depending on your circumstances, such as dietary restrictions or special conditions, you may have different goals. Common nutritional goals include:

- Getting enough folate, iron, and calcium.
- Ensuring a variety of fruits and vegetables.
- Including lean protein sources.
- Incorporating healthy fats.
- Maintaining proper hydration.

Step 2: Plan Your Meals

- Aim for three main meals (breakfast, lunch, dinner) and healthy snacks between meals.
- Choose a variety of foods to meet your nutritional goals.

- Include a source of protein, a serving of whole grains, and plenty of fruits and vegetables in each meal.
- Incorporate dairy or fortified plant-based milk for calcium.
- Plan snacks that include protein and fiber to keep you satisfied.

Step 3: Sample Meal Ideas

Here are some meal ideas to inspire your planning:

Breakfast:
- A parfait of Greek yogurt, granola, and berries.
- Oatmeal topped with nuts, seeds, and sliced banana.
- Whole-grain bread with spinach scrambled eggs.

Lunch:
- Quinoa salad with mixed vegetables and a tahini dressing.
- Whole-grain bread toasted with turkey and avocado.
- A side of mixed greens and lentil soup.

Dinner:
- Steamed broccoli and baked salmon served with quinoa.
- Stir-fried tofu with brown rice and a variety of vegetables.
- grilled chicken paired with asparagus and sweet potatoes.

Snacks:
- Apple slices with almond butter.
- Baby carrots with hummus.
- Greek yogurt topped with a mixture of almonds and honey.

Step 4: Plan and Prep

-Based on your meal plan, create a grocery list.
- Shop for fresh ingredients, and consider purchasing items for the entire week to reduce the need for frequent trips to the store.
- Set aside time for meal prep, such as washing and chopping vegetables, cooking grains, and preparing some meals in advance.

Step 5: Stay Hydrated

-To stay hydrated during the day, sip lots of water. You can also include herbal teas or infused water for variety.

Step 6: Monitor Your Weight

- Keep track of your weight gain during pregnancy to ensure it's within the recommended range. Your healthcare provider can guide you on this.

Step 7: Adjust as Needed

- Be flexible with your meal plan. If you experience food aversions, nausea, or other issues, adapt your plan to what you can comfortably eat.

Remember that it's important to consult with your healthcare provider or a registered dietitian to tailor your meal plan to your specific needs. They can provide guidance on the best choices for you and your baby.

Meal planning during pregnancy can help you maintain a healthy and well-balanced diet that supports both your well-being and the development of your baby.

BALANCED MEALS FOR EACH TRIMESTER

Creating balanced meals for each trimester of pregnancy is important because your nutritional needs change as your baby grows. Here are some general guidelines for balanced meals during each trimester:

First Trimester (Weeks 1-12):

During the first trimester, your baby's organs are forming, and you may experience morning sickness. Focus on easy-to-digest foods and staying hydrated. A balanced meal might include:

- Breakfast: A glass of water and oatmeal with berries.
- Lunch: a mixed green salad and grilled chicken breast.
- Snack: Greek yogurt and a handful of almonds.
- Dinner: baked salmon served over quinoa and steaming broccoli.
- Snack: Sliced apples with peanut butter.

Second Trimester (Weeks 13-27):

This is your baby's time of fast growth.. Aim for nutrient-dense foods to support this development. A balanced meal might include:

- Breakfast: toasted whole-grain bread with scrambled eggs with spinach.
- Lunch: mixed vegetable quinoa salad with tahini dressing.
- Snack: Carrots and hummus.
- Dinner: Stir-fried tofu with brown rice and a variety of vegetables.
- Snack: A piece of fruit and a small handful of walnuts.

Third Trimester (Weeks 28-40):

In the final trimester, your baby continues to grow, and you need extra calories and nutrients. Include foods rich in iron and calcium for healthy development. A balanced meal might include:

- Breakfast: Greek yogurt parfait with berries, granola, and a glass of milk.
- Lunch: On whole-grain bread, a turkey and avocado sandwich is served with a side salad.
- Snack: Sliced bell peppers with guacamole.
- Dinner: Grilled steak with sweet potato and asparagus.
- Snack: Cottage cheese with pineapple.

General Tips for All Trimesters:

1. Stay well-hydrated. Drink plenty of water throughout the day.

2. Include a source of protein in each meal, such as lean meats, tofu, legumes, or dairy products.

3. Prioritize fruits and vegetables to get a variety of vitamins and minerals.

4. Incorporate whole grains like brown rice, quinoa, and whole-grain bread for sustained energy.

5. Include healthy fats from sources like avocados, nuts, and olive oil.

6. Monitor your weight gain to ensure it's within the recommended range. Seek advice from your healthcare provider.

7. Listen to your body and adapt your meals to any food aversions or cravings you may experience.

Remember that every pregnancy is unique, and individual needs can vary. It's important to consult with your healthcare provider or a registered dietitian to create a personalized meal plan that considers your specific circumstances and health. They can provide tailored guidance to ensure a healthy and balanced diet throughout your pregnancy.

SNACKS AND HEALTHY OPTIONS

Healthy Snack Options During Pregnancy

Choosing healthy snacks during pregnancy can help you maintain your energy levels, manage hunger, and provide the essential nutrients your body and your baby need. Here are some nutritious snack options:

1. **Fresh Fruit:**
   - Sliced apples, oranges, berries, or a banana can provide vitamins, fiber, and a natural energy boost.

2. **Greek Yogurt:**
   - Greek yogurt is abundant in protein and calcium. For sweetness, add some honey or fresh fruit.

3. **Nuts and Seeds:**

- Almonds, walnuts, chia seeds, or flaxseeds are packed with healthy fats, protein, and fiber.

4. **Hummus and Veggies:**
   - Dip carrot sticks, cucumber slices, or bell pepper strips in hummus for a satisfying and nutritious snack.

5. **Cottage Cheese:**
   - Cottage cheese is high in protein and calcium. Top it with fresh pineapple, peaches, or a drizzle of honey.

6. **String Cheese:**
   - String cheese is a convenient source of calcium and protein. It's a great on-the-go option.

7. **Hard-Boiled Eggs:**
   - Hard-boiled eggs are a portable source of protein. Sprinkle with a pinch of salt or pepper for flavor.

8. **Whole-Grain Crackers:**
   - Pair whole-grain crackers with a slice of lean turkey or a small amount of low-fat cheese.

9. **Oatmeal:**
   - A small bowl of oatmeal with a touch of honey or fresh berries is a filling and nutritious snack.

10. **Smoothies:**

- Blend a smoothie with Greek yogurt, fresh fruit, spinach, and a splash of milk for a refreshing and nutrient-packed snack.

11. **Popcorn:**
   - Air-popped popcorn is a low-calorie whole-grain snack. Season with a sprinkle of nutritional yeast or your favorite spices.

12. **Dried Fruits:**
   - Dried fruits like apricots, figs, and raisins provide natural sweetness and energy. Be mindful of portion sizes due to their calorie density.

13. **Avocado Toast:**
   - Spread ripe avocado on whole-grain toast and add a dash of salt or pepper for a satisfying snack.

14. **Cereal with Milk:**
   - Opt for a whole-grain cereal with low-fat or fortified plant-based milk for a quick and easy snack.

15. **Rice Cakes:**
   - Top rice cakes with almond butter and sliced banana for a crunchy and satisfying treat.

16. **Frozen Grapes:**
   - Frozen grapes are a sweet and refreshing option for a hot day.

When choosing snacks, aim for a combination of macronutrients (protein, carbohydrates, and healthy fats) to keep you feeling full and satisfied. Additionally, focus on portion control to avoid excessive calorie intake. It's important to listen to your body and eat when you're hungry, as pregnancy can lead to varying appetite levels.

Remember that individual dietary needs can differ, so consulting with your healthcare provider or a registered dietitian can help you create a personalized snack plan that addresses your unique requirements and preferences during pregnancy.

REAL FOOD RECIPES FOR PREGNANCY

Here are a few nutritious and delicious real food recipes suitable for pregnancy:

1. Quinoa and Black Bean Salad:
   - Ingredients:
     - 1 cup quinoa
     - 2 cups water
     - 1 can black beans, drained and rinsed
     - 1 cup frozen or fresh corn
     - 1 red bell pepper, diced
     - A quarter cup of red onion, chopped finely
     - 1/4 cup fresh cilantro, chopped
     - Juice of 2 limes
     - 2 tablespoons olive oil
     - Salt and pepper to taste

- Instructions:
    1. Rinse quinoa in a fine-mesh strainer. In a saucepan, bring quinoa and water to a boil, then reduce heat, cover, and simmer for 15 minutes or until cooked.
    2. In a large bowl, combine cooked quinoa, black beans, corn, red pepper, red onion, and cilantro.
    3. In a small mixing bowl, combine the lime juice, olive oil, salt, and pepper. Mix the salad by tossing it with the dressing. Serve chilled.

2. Sweet Potato and Chickpea Curry:
   - Ingredients:
    - 2 medium peeled and sliced sweet potatoes
       - 1 can drained and rinsed chickpeas
       - 1 onion, diced
       - 2 cloves garlic, minced
       - 1 can diced tomatoes
       - 1 can coconut milk
       - 2 tablespoons curry powder
       - 1 teaspoon ground turmeric
       - Salt and pepper to taste
       - Fresh cilantro for garnish
       - Cooked brown rice or quinoa (optional, for serving)

   - Instructions:
    1. In a large pot, sauté the onion and garlic in a little oil until softened.

2. Add the sweet potatoes, chickpeas, diced tomatoes, and coconut milk.

3. Stir in the curry powder, turmeric, salt, and pepper. Bring to a simmer and continue to boil until the sweet potatoes are cooked.

4. Serve over cooked brown rice or quinoa, garnished with fresh cilantro.

3. Salmon with Asparagus and Quinoa:
  - Ingredients:
    - 2 salmon fillets
    - 1 bunch of asparagus, trimmed
    - 1 cup quinoa
    - 2 tablespoons olive oil
    - 1 lemon, zested and juiced
    - Salt and pepper to taste

  - Instructions:
    1. Set the oven's temperature to 400 degrees Fahrenheit, or 200 degrees Celsius.

2. Place the salmon fillets and trimmed asparagus on a baking sheet. Add a drizzle of olive oil and taste-test salt and pepper for seasoning.

3. Roast for 15-20 minutes or until salmon flakes easily and asparagus is tender.

4. Meanwhile, cook quinoa according to package instructions.

5. Serve the salmon and asparagus over a bed of quinoa, drizzle with lemon juice.

These recipes are rich in essential nutrients and provide a variety of flavors to keep your meals exciting during pregnancy. They also offer a good balance of carbohydrates, protein, healthy fats, and fiber to support your nutritional needs. Remember to consult with your healthcare provider or a registered dietitian for personalized dietary guidance during your pregnancy.

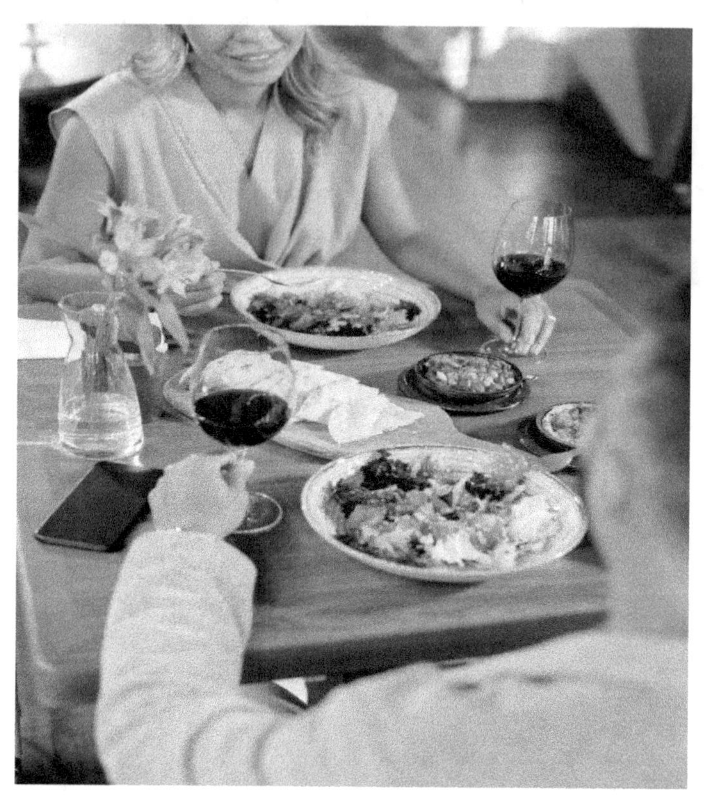

CHAPTER FOUR

MANAGING COMMON PREGNANCY SYMPTOMS

Pregnancy can bring about a variety of symptoms and discomforts. While these experiences can differ from person to person, here are some tips to help manage common pregnancy symptoms:

1. **Morning Sickness:**
   - Eat modest, frequent meals throughout the day to keep blood sugar levels steady.
   - Stay hydrated by sipping on clear fluids like water or ginger tea.
   - Ginger, either in tea, capsules, or candies, may help alleviate nausea.
   - Consider vitamin B6 supplements (under the guidance of a healthcare provider).

2. **Fatigue:**
   - Get enough of sleep and pay attention to your body. Take naps as needed.
   - Prioritize a healthy, balanced diet to maintain your energy levels.
   - Light exercise, like walking, can help reduce fatigue.

3. **Heartburn and Indigestion:**

- Eat smaller meals and avoid heavy or spicy foods.
   - Consume your last meal a few hours before bedtime.
   - Prop your upper body up with pillows while sleeping.
   - Over-the-counter antacids might help, but before taking them, speak with your doctor.

4. **Constipation:**
   - Include high-fiber foods in your diet, like whole grains, fruits, and vegetables.
   - - To stay well hydrated, sip lots of water.
   - Light exercise can also help improve digestion.

5. **Swelling and Water Retention:**
   - Avoid excessive salt intake.
   - Elevate your legs whenever possible.
   - Stay active, but be sure to rest and put your feet up when needed.

6. **Back Pain:**
   - Maintain good posture to reduce strain on your back.
   - Wear comfortable, supportive shoes.
   - Gentle exercises, such as prenatal yoga or swimming, can help alleviate back pain.
   - Consider a prenatal massage or physical therapy if pain is severe.

7. **Leg Cramps:**
   - Stay hydrated.

- Stretch your calf muscles regularly.
- Eat foods high in potassium, such as bananas, as part of your diet.
- Talk to your healthcare provider about safe magnesium supplementation.

8. **Insomnia:**
- Create a relaxing bedtime routine, which may include a warm bath or soothing music.
- Maintain a cool, dark bedroom.
- Use extra pillows to support your body and find a comfortable sleep position.

9. **Mood Swings:**
- Discuss your feelings with a mental health professional, your pals, or your partner.
- Use calming strategies like mindfulness and deep breathing.
- Maintain a well-balanced diet to support mood stability.

10. **Frequent Urination:**
- Limit caffeine intake.
- Stay hydrated but reduce fluid consumption close to bedtime.
- Before you turn in for the night, empty your bladder.

Remember that every pregnancy is unique, and it's important to consult your healthcare provider if you're experiencing severe or persistent symptoms. They can provide tailored guidance and recommend appropriate remedies or treatments to manage your specific pregnancy-related discomforts.

NAUSEA AND MORNING SICKNESS

During pregnancy, nausea and morning sickness are common symptoms, particularly in the first trimester. While they can be uncomfortable, there are several strategies to help manage these symptoms:

1. **Eat Small, Frequent Meals:**
   - Instead of three large meals, opt for six smaller meals throughout the day. An empty stomach can exacerbate nausea.

2. **Stay Hydrated:**
   - Sip on clear fluids like water, ginger tea, or electrolyte drinks to prevent dehydration.

3. **Ginger:**
   - Ginger, in various forms, such as ginger tea, ginger candies, or ginger supplements, can help alleviate nausea for many people.

4. **Avoid Trigger Foods:**
   - Identify and avoid foods that trigger your nausea. Foods that are oily, spicy, or have strong aromas are frequently the culprits.

5. **Vitamin B6:**
   - Under the guidance of your healthcare provider, consider vitamin B6 supplements, as they may help reduce nausea.

6. **Acupressure Wristbands:**
   - Some pregnant individuals find relief from nausea using acupressure wristbands, like Sea-Bands.

7. **Aromatherapy:**
   - Scents like lemon, peppermint, or lavender may help ease nausea. You can use essential oils or inhale fresh slices of lemon.

8. **Rest:**
   - Fatigue can worsen nausea, so prioritize rest and take naps if needed.

9. **Avoid Triggers:**
   - Identify and avoid smells or sights that trigger your nausea.

10. **Prescription Medication:**
   - In severe cases, your healthcare provider may recommend prescription medications to manage morning sickness. They must only be used under a physician's guidance.

11. **Mindful Eating:**
   - Chew your meal well and slowly while   eating. Avoid rushing through meals.

12. **Cold Foods:**
   - Sometimes, cold or room-temperature foods are better tolerated than hot foods.

13. **Distract Yourself:**
   - Engage in activities that can divert your attention from nausea, such as reading, watching TV, or going for a short walk.

It's important to note that morning sickness usually improves as you enter the second trimester. However, if your symptoms are severe, persistent, or if you're unable to keep any food or fluids down, it's essential to consult your healthcare provider. They can provide guidance, monitor your condition, and recommend appropriate treatments to ensure both your and your baby's health.

HEARTBURN AND INDIGESTION

Heartburn and indigestion are common discomforts during pregnancy, especially in the second and third trimesters when the growing uterus can put pressure on the stomach. The following are some methods to help control and lessen these symptoms:

1. **Smaller, More Frequent Meals:**

  - To ease the strain on your stomach, choose smaller, more frequent meals rather than larger ones.

2. **Stay Upright After Eating:**
   Steer clear of lying down right after eating. Give your body time to digest food by staying upright for at least 1-2 hours after eating.

3. **Avoid Trigger Foods:**
   - Identify foods that trigger heartburn and indigestion for you. Common triggers include spicy, greasy, or acidic foods.

4. **Proper Meal Timing:**
   - Have your last meal of the day a few hours before bedtime to reduce nighttime symptoms.

5. **Elevate Your Upper Body:**
   - Use extra pillows to elevate your upper body while sleeping. This can help prevent stomach acid from flowing back into your esophagus.

6. **Wear Loose-Fitting Clothing:**
   - Tight clothing can put additional pressure on your abdomen. Opt for loose-fitting attire.

7. **Chew Gum:**
   - Chewing sugarless gum after a meal can stimulate saliva production, which can help neutralize stomach acid.

8. **Avoid Smoking:**
   - If you smoke, consider quitting. Smoking can contribute to heartburn and indigestion.

9. **Antacids:**
   - Temporary relief can be obtained with over-the-counter antacids such as Rolaids or Tums. However, consult your healthcare provider before using them regularly.

10. **Papaya Enzymes:**
   - Some individuals find relief from papaya enzyme supplements. Speak with your doctor before attempting them.

11. **Ginger Tea:**
   - Ginger tea can help soothe the digestive system and reduce discomfort.

12. **Proton Pump Inhibitors (PPIs) or H2 Blockers:**
   - In more severe cases, your healthcare provider may prescribe medications like PPIs or H2 blockers to reduce stomach acid production. Only medical supervision is recommended when using them.

13. **Consult Your Healthcare Provider:**
   - If heartburn and indigestion are persistent, severe, or interfere with your daily life, consult your healthcare provider. They are able to provide direction and suggest suitable interventions.

Remember that heartburn and indigestion are common during pregnancy, and they usually improve after giving birth. In the meantime, these strategies can help you manage the discomfort and alleviate symptoms. If your symptoms are severe or concerning, do not hesitate to seek guidance from your healthcare provider.

CONSTIPATION AND DIGESTIVE HEALTH

Constipation is a common issue during pregnancy, primarily due to hormonal changes, pressure on the digestive tract, and iron supplements. To promote digestive health and relieve constipation during pregnancy, consider these strategies:

1. **Fiber-Rich Diet:**
   - Increase your fiber intake by including more whole grains, fruits, vegetables, and legumes in your diet. Fiber helps soften stool and promote regular bowel movements.

2. **Stay Hydrated:**
   - Stay hydrated throughout the day to maintain soft, passable stools.

3. **Prunes or Prune Juice:**
   - Prunes are well-known for having a laxative effect on their own. Consider eating a few prunes or drinking prune juice to alleviate constipation.

4. **Exercise:**

   - Gentle physical activity, such as walking or swimming, can help stimulate your bowels and improve digestion.

5. **Probiotics:**
   - Probiotic-rich foods like yogurt and kefir can promote healthy gut bacteria and help regulate bowel movements.

6. **Avoid Iron Supplements on an Empty Stomach:**
   - If you're taking iron supplements, take them with a small snack or meal to reduce their potential to cause constipation.

7. **Psyllium Husk:**
   - Psyllium husk, available as a dietary supplement, can help bulk up stools and improve bowel regularity. Ensure you consult with your healthcare provider before using supplements.

8. **Limit Iron Supplements When Possible:**
   - If your healthcare provider agrees, you may be able to reduce the dose of iron supplements or switch to a different type with fewer side effects.

9. **Consult Your Healthcare Provider:**
   - If constipation is persistent, severe, or accompanied by other concerning symptoms, consult your healthcare provider. They can recommend safe laxatives or medications suitable for pregnancy.

10. **Stool Softeners:**
   - Some pregnant individuals may benefit from over-the-counter stool softeners like docusate sodium. Be sure to speak with your doctor before taking any medications.

It's important to address constipation during pregnancy, as chronic constipation can lead to hemorrhoids or worsen preexisting hemorrhoids. Additionally, it's essential to rule out any underlying digestive issues. Always consult with your healthcare provider before making significant dietary changes or using medications, even if they are over-the-counter.

Maintaining good digestive health and regular bowel movements is crucial during pregnancy, not only to alleviate discomfort but also to ensure the well-being of both you and your baby.

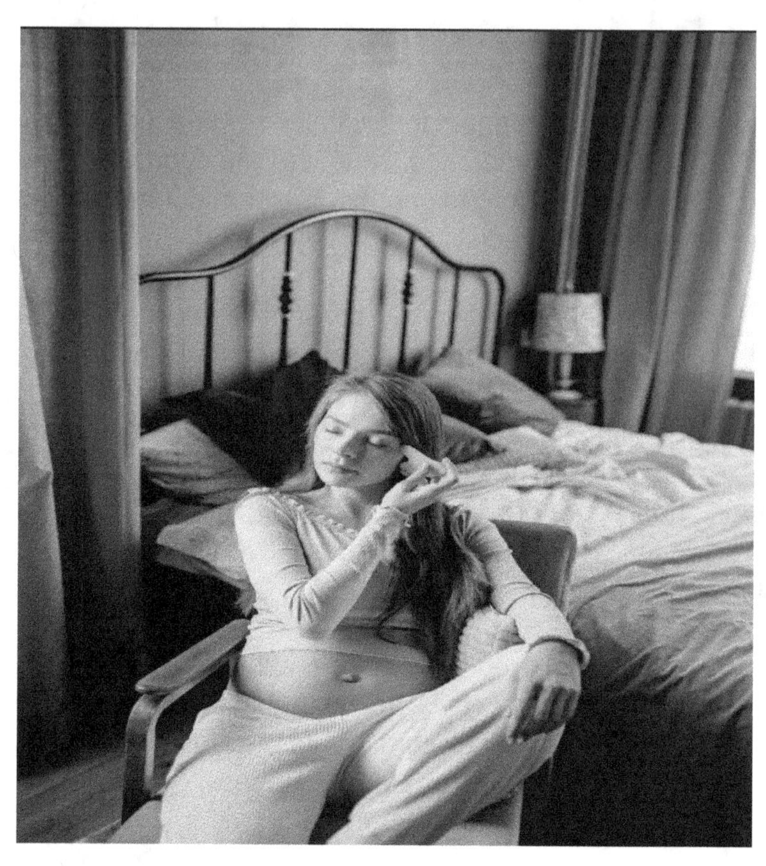

CHAPTER FIVE

STAYING ACTIVE AND FIT

Staying active and fit during pregnancy is important for your physical and emotional well-being, as well as the health of your baby. Here are some guidelines for maintaining an active and safe exercise routine during pregnancy:

1. **Consult Your Healthcare Provider:**
   - See your healthcare practitioner prior to beginning or extending an exercise regimen while you are pregnant. They can provide guidance based on your specific medical history and pregnancy.

2. **Choose Low-Impact Activities:**
   - Opt for low-impact exercises that are easier on your joints and the growing baby, such as walking, swimming, stationary cycling, and prenatal yoga.

3. **Warm Up and Cool Down:**
   - Always start your exercise routine with a warm-up to prepare your body, and end with a cool-down to gradually lower your heart rate.

4. **Stay Hydrated:**
   - Stay hydrated by sipping lots of water prior to, during, and following activity.

5. **Wear Proper Clothing:**
   - Choose comfortable and breathable workout attire that provides support.

6. **Listen to Your Body:**
   - Observe your feelings while exercising. If you feel any pain, lightheadedness, dyspnea, or other discomfort, stop right away and get help from your doctor.

7. **Avoid Overexertion:**
   - While it's important to stay active, avoid pushing yourself to exhaustion. Modify your exercise routine to match your energy levels and any physical changes.

8. **Focus on Core and Pelvic Floor:**
   - Incorporate exercises to strengthen your core and pelvic floor, such as Kegels, as they can help support your growing belly and reduce the risk of issues like incontinence.

9. **Maintain Good Posture:**
   - Pay attention to your posture during exercise to reduce the risk of back pain. Engage your core muscles and avoid exercises that strain your back.

10. **Prenatal Classes:**
    - Consider attending prenatal fitness classes led by instructors trained to work with pregnant

individuals. These classes are tailored to your specific needs.

11. **Balance and Stability:**
   - As your body changes, your balance may be affected. Be cautious when doing exercises that require balance, and use support when necessary.

12. **Strengthening and Stretching:**
   - Include a mix of strength training and stretching exercises to improve flexibility and muscle tone.

13. **Avoid High-Risk Activities:**
   - Steer clear of activities with a high risk of falling or injury, such as contact sports, skiing, and horseback riding.

14. **Postpartum Planning:**
   - Think about your postpartum fitness plan. After giving birth, gradually ease back into exercise under the guidance of your healthcare provider.

Remember that every pregnancy is unique, and your exercise routine should be tailored to your individual circumstances. Stay in communication with your healthcare provider, who can provide guidance and monitor your progress throughout your pregnancy. Staying active and fit can help you manage pregnancy discomfort, maintain a healthy weight, and prepare your body for labor and delivery.

YOGA AND GENTLE WORKOUTS

Yoga and gentle workouts can be excellent choices for maintaining physical and mental well-being during pregnancy. These activities offer numerous benefits, including improved flexibility, relaxation, and stress reduction. Here are some considerations for practicing yoga and gentle workouts during pregnancy:

1. Prenatal Yoga:
   - Prenatal yoga classes are specifically designed to address the needs and comfort of pregnant individuals. They focus on gentle stretching, breathing, and relaxation techniques.

2. Consult Your Healthcare Provider:
   - Before starting or continuing any exercise routine during pregnancy, including yoga, consult with your healthcare provider to ensure it's safe for your specific situation.

3. Find Experienced Instructors:
   - Look for yoga instructors who are experienced in teaching prenatal yoga. They can provide guidance on modifications and postures suitable for each trimester.

4. Gentle Workouts:
   - Consider gentle workouts like walking, swimming, stationary cycling, or Pilates. These

exercises can help you maintain fitness without putting excessive strain on your body.

5. Listen to Your Body:
   - Pay close attention to how you feel during yoga or workouts. If you experience discomfort, dizziness, or pain, stop immediately and modify the activity as needed.

6. Avoid Overexertion:
   - Be mindful not to overexert yourself. Modify your yoga or workout routine to match your energy levels and changing physical conditions.

7. Stay Hydrated:
   - Drink plenty of water to stay well-hydrated during and after your yoga or workout sessions.

8. Modify Poses:
   - As your pregnancy goes on, adjust your yoga poses. Steer clear of inversions, deep twists, and postures that compress the abdomen. Focus on gentle stretches and relaxation.

9. Practice Breathing Techniques:
   - Incorporate deep breathing and relaxation techniques to reduce stress and promote overall well-being

10. Posture and Alignment:

- Pay attention to your posture and body alignment during yoga and gentle workouts to avoid straining your back or pelvis.

11. Supportive Attire:
   - Wear comfortable, breathable workout attire that provides support for your growing body.

12. Balance and Stability:
   - As your balance may be affected by your changing body, use props or support as needed to maintain stability during yoga or workouts.

13. Prenatal Fitness Classes:
   - Consider participating in prenatal fitness classes that are specifically tailored to the needs of pregnant individuals. These classes can provide a supportive and social environment.

Yoga and gentle workouts can help you stay active and maintain your physical and mental well-being during pregnancy. They can also prepare your body for labor and postpartum recovery. Always prioritize safety and consult with your healthcare provider to ensure that your chosen activities are suitable for your pregnancy.

STAYING MOTIVATED

Staying motivated to maintain a healthy lifestyle during pregnancy can be a challenge, but it's essential for your well-being and the health of your baby. To help you stay motivated, consider these tips:

1. **Set Clear Goals:** Define specific and realistic health and fitness goals for your pregnancy. Setting and maintaining clear goals will keep you motivated and focused.

2. **Create a Routine:** Establish a daily or weekly routine that includes exercise, healthy eating, and self-care. A consistent schedule makes it easier to stick to your plan.

3. **Find Enjoyable Activities:** Choose exercises and activities that you genuinely enjoy. Whether it's prenatal yoga, swimming, walking, or dancing, having fun will make it easier to stay motivated.

4. **Enlist a Workout Buddy:** If possible, find a workout partner who can join you in your fitness routine. It's often more enjoyable and motivating when you have someone to share the experience with.

5. **Join Prenatal Fitness Classes:** Consider participating in prenatal fitness classes or groups. You'll meet other pregnant individuals and receive guidance and motivation from instructors.

6. **Track Your Progress:** Keep a journal or use a fitness app to track your progress. Observing progress can serve as a powerful incentive.

7. **Reward Yourself:** Set up a rewards system for meeting your goals. When you accomplish a goal, reward yourself with something exceptional.

8. **Stay Informed:** Educate yourself about the benefits of a healthy lifestyle during pregnancy. Understanding how it positively impacts you and your baby can be a powerful motivator.

9. **Listen to Your Body:** Be attuned to your body's signals. If you're tired or experiencing discomfort, it's okay to take a break. Prioritizing the health of both you and your child is essential.

10. **Stay Positive:** Maintain a positive attitude and focus on the positive changes happening in your body. A positive mindset can be a significant source of motivation.

11. **Seek Support:** Share your goals with friends and family who can provide support and encouragement. Sometimes, a supportive network can make a significant difference.

12. **Consult with Experts:** Regularly consult with your healthcare provider and consider working with a fitness professional or a nutritionist who

specializes in prenatal care. Their guidance can help you stay on track.

13. **Visualize Your Baby:** Imagine the health benefits that your baby will gain from your healthy lifestyle. Visualizing a happy, healthy baby can provide a strong incentive.

14. **Stay Flexible:** Be adaptable with your goals and routine. Pregnancy comes with changes and fluctuations, so it's important to adjust your expectations when needed.

15. **Self-Care:** Prioritize self-care, including adequate rest and stress management. Reducing stress and getting enough sleep can help you stay motivated.

Remember that motivation can ebb and flow, and it's perfectly normal to have days when you feel less enthusiastic. The key is to stay consistent and keep your long-term health and the well-being of your baby in mind. If you ever struggle with motivation, don't hesitate to reach out to your support network, healthcare provider, or a counselor for guidance and encouragement.

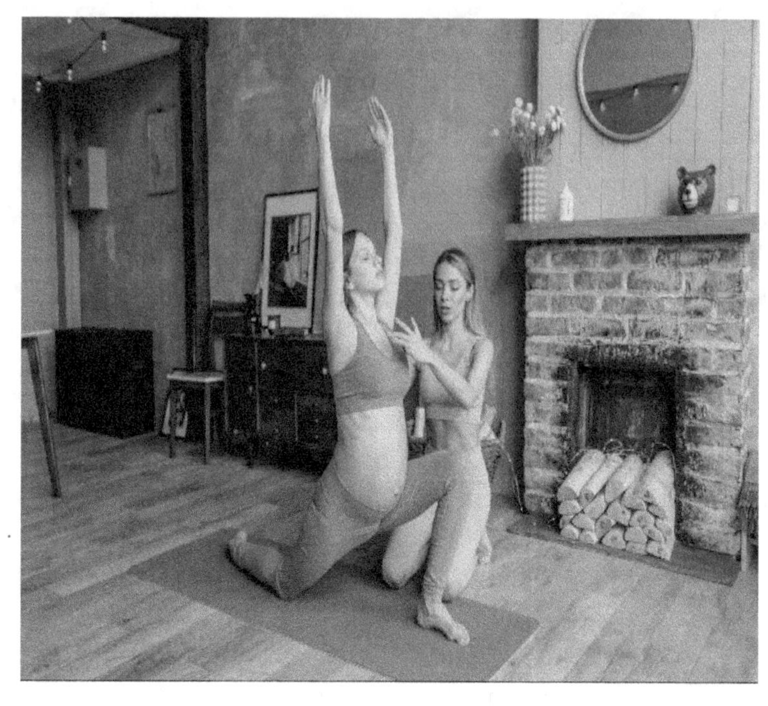

CHAPTER SIX

SPECIAL DIETARY CONSIDERATION

During pregnancy, certain dietary considerations become especially important to ensure the health and well-being of both you and your developing baby. Here are some special dietary considerations for pregnant individuals:

1. Folate and Folic Acid:
   - Folate is crucial for preventing neural tube defects in the baby. Eat foods high in folate, such as legumes, leafy greens, and fortified cereals. A folic acid supplement may also be suggested by your healthcare provider.

2. Iron:
   - Iron is essential for preventing anemia and supporting your baby's growth. Consume iron-rich foods like lean meats, poultry, fish, and fortified cereals. If needed, your healthcare provider may suggest iron supplements.

3. Calcium:
   - Calcium is necessary for your baby's bone development. Include dairy products, fortified plant-based milk, tofu, and leafy greens in your diet to meet your calcium needs.

4. DHA (Omega-3 Fatty Acid):
   - The development of your baby's brain and eyes depends on DHA. Include sources of DHA in your diet, such as fatty fish (like salmon and trout) or consider a DHA supplement.

5. Hydration:
   - Staying hydrated is vital during pregnancy. Sip on lots of water, herbal teas, and other clear beverages. Dehydration can lead to preterm contractions and other complications.

6. Protein:
   - Protein supports your baby's growth. Incorporate foods such as dairy, almonds, beans, fish, poultry, eggs, and lean meats into your diet.

7. Fiber:
   - Dietary fiber can help alleviate constipation, a common issue during pregnancy. Consume whole grains, fruits, and vegetables for a fiber-rich diet.

8. Limit Caffeine and Alcohol:
   - Avoiding excessive alcohol and caffeine consumption is advised. Limit caffeine to 200-300 mg per day and eliminate alcohol during pregnancy.

9. Food Safety:
   - Pay attention to food safety. Steer clear of raw or undercooked meats, eggs, and seafood. Be cautious with unpasteurized dairy products and deli

meats, as they can carry the risk of foodborne illnesses.

10. Weight Gain:
   - Monitor your weight gain during pregnancy. It's essential to gain an appropriate amount of weight to support your baby's development without excessive gain.

11. Balanced Diet:
   - Strive for a diet that is well-balanced and comprises a range of dietary groups. This ensures you receive essential nutrients.

12. Food Aversions and Cravings:
   - Be flexible with your diet due to potential food aversions and cravings. As long as your overall diet remains balanced and nutritious, occasional indulgences are okay.

13. Nutrient Supplements:
   - Follow your healthcare provider's recommendations for taking prenatal vitamins and supplements, as they can help fill nutritional gaps.

14. Special Dietary Needs:
   - If you have specific dietary restrictions or medical conditions (e.g., gestational diabetes), work closely with a registered dietitian to plan a suitable and safe diet.

15. Gestational Diabetes:

- If you develop gestational diabetes, carefully manage your blood sugar levels through dietary modifications, physical activity, and, if necessary, medications.

It's important to consult with your healthcare provider or a registered dietitian to create a personalized dietary plan that addresses your unique needs during pregnancy. A well-balanced and nutrient-rich diet is key to supporting the healthy growth and development of your baby while ensuring your own well-being.

VEGETARIAN AND VEGAN PREGNANCY

Maintaining a vegetarian or vegan diet during pregnancy is entirely possible and can be a healthy choice for you and your baby. However, it requires careful planning to ensure you get all the essential nutrients. Here are some considerations for a vegetarian or vegan pregnancy:

1. Protein:
   - Consume a variety of plant-based protein sources such as legumes (lentils, chickpeas), tofu, tempeh, quinoa, and nuts. Including a combination of these foods can help you meet your protein needs.

2. Iron:

- Plant-based sources of iron include dark leafy greens, fortified cereals, beans, and lentils. Pair iron-rich foods with vitamin C-rich foods (e.g., citrus fruits, bell peppers) to enhance iron absorption.

3. Calcium:
- Include calcium-rich foods like fortified plant-based milk, tofu, tahini, and leafy greens in your diet. If needed, consider calcium-fortified supplements.

4. Vitamin B12:
- Vitamin B12 is not naturally found in plant-based foods, so it's essential to take a B12 supplement or consume B12-fortified foods. To find out the right dosage for supplements, speak with your healthcare professional.

5. Omega-3 Fatty Acids:
- Include sources of plant-based omega-3s like flaxseeds, chia seeds, and walnuts. You can also consider algae-based DHA supplements.

6. Folate:
- Eat foods high in folate, such as legumes, leafy greens, and cereals with added folate. If necessary, take a folic acid supplement as recommended by your healthcare provider.

7. Protein Combinations:

   - Complement proteins by combining different plant-based sources, such as beans and rice, to ensure you get a complete amino acid profile.

8. Fiber:
   - A vegetarian or vegan diet is often rich in fiber, which can help alleviate constipation, a common pregnancy symptom.

9. Vitamin D:
   - Ensure you get enough sun exposure for vitamin D or consider a vitamin D supplement if recommended by your healthcare provider.

10. Hydration:
   - Sip plenty of water and herbal teas to stay hydrated.

11. Snacking:
   - Plan for healthy snacks throughout the day to meet your nutritional needs and manage hunger.

12. Monitor Weight Gain:
   - Keep track of your weight gain to ensure it falls within recommended guidelines.

13. Consult a Registered Dietitian:
   - Consider consulting a registered dietitian or nutritionist who specializes in vegetarian and vegan diets to create a balanced and nutrient-rich meal plan.

14. Food Safety:
   - Be aware of food safety, avoiding unpasteurized dairy products and practicing proper food handling to reduce the risk of foodborne illnesses.

15. Nutrient Supplements:
   - Follow your healthcare provider's recommendations for taking prenatal vitamins and supplements, which may include additional iron, calcium, or other nutrients.

It's crucial to plan your diet carefully to ensure you receive all the necessary nutrients for a healthy pregnancy. A well-balanced vegetarian or vegan diet can be not only safe but also a nutritious and fulfilling choice during pregnancy. Always consult with your healthcare provider and consider seeking guidance from a registered dietitian to create a personalized dietary plan.

FOOD ALLERGIES AND SENSITIVITIES

If you have food allergies or sensitivities, managing your diet during pregnancy is particularly important. Here are some guidelines for handling food allergies and sensitivities during pregnancy:

1. Identify and Avoid Allergenic Foods:
   - If you have known food allergies, continue to avoid the specific allergenic foods that trigger your

reactions. Peanuts, tree nuts, dairy, eggs, soy, wheat, fish, and shellfish are among the common allergies.

2. Consult an Allergist:
   - If you're unsure about potential food allergies, consult with an allergist or immunologist for allergy testing.

3. Read Labels Carefully:
   - When shopping for food, read labels diligently to identify allergenic ingredients and potential cross-contamination.

4. Communicate with Restaurants:
   - When dining out, inform restaurant staff about your food allergies and ask about their procedures for avoiding cross-contact.

5. Allergy-Free Alternatives:
   - Seek out allergy-free alternatives and substitutes for foods you can't consume. Many allergy-friendly products are available in stores.

6. Plan Balanced Meals:
   - Plan balanced meals that accommodate your dietary restrictions. You may need to be creative in finding suitable protein sources and nutrients.

7. Consult a Dietitian:
   - Consider working with a registered dietitian or nutritionist who specializes in allergies and

sensitivities to help you plan a well-rounded diet that meets your nutritional needs.

8. Nutrient Supplements:
   - If your dietary restrictions limit your intake of essential nutrients, your healthcare provider may recommend supplements to fill the gaps.

9. Monitor for Cross-Contamination:
   - Be vigilant about cross-contamination when preparing food at home. Use separate utensils, cutting boards, and cooking surfaces to avoid allergen exposure.

10. Medications and Allergies:
   - Discuss any medications, including antihistamines or epinephrine auto-injectors, with your healthcare provider. Ensure you have your prescribed medications readily available in case of accidental exposure.

11. Seek Medical Attention:
   - If you experience an allergic reaction, seek immediate medical attention, especially if the symptoms are severe or involve difficulty breathing, swelling, or anaphylaxis.

12. Food Sensitivities:
   - If you have food sensitivities, avoid or limit the specific foods that trigger your sensitivities. Work with a healthcare provider or dietitian to ensure you

meet your nutritional needs while accommodating your sensitivities.

It's crucial to communicate your food allergies and sensitivities to your healthcare provider so they can provide guidance and support throughout your pregnancy. Managing your dietary restrictions while ensuring you and your baby receive the necessary nutrients is possible with careful planning and proper precautions.

GESTATIONAL DIABETES AND REAL FOOD MANAGEMENT

Managing gestational diabetes through a real food approach involves making dietary choices that prioritize whole, unprocessed foods and managing carbohydrate intake. Here are some guidelines for managing gestational diabetes through real food:

1. Balanced Meals:
   - Strive for meals that are well-balanced and contain a mix of healthy fats, protein, and carbs. Whole grains, lean proteins, and non-starchy vegetables should be staples in your diet.

2. Whole Grains:
   - Choose whole grains like quinoa, brown rice, and whole wheat pasta over refined grains to help stabilize blood sugar levels.

3. Carbohydrate Control:

- Monitor your carbohydrate intake by paying attention to portion sizes and choosing carbohydrates with a lower glycemic index (GI). Low-GI foods are less likely to cause rapid spikes in blood sugar.

4. Fiber-Rich Foods:
- Include high-fiber foods like vegetables, legumes, and fruits (in moderation) in your diet to help manage blood sugar levels.

5. Lean Proteins:
- Incorporate lean sources of protein like poultry, fish, tofu, and beans into your meals. In addition to keeping your blood sugar stable, protein can help you feel full.

6. Healthy Fats:
- Choose healthy fats from sources like almonds, avocados, and olive oil. These fats can help control blood sugar and promote overall health.

7. Sugar Avoidance:
- Avoid processed foods and drinks that have added sugar. These may result in sharp rises in blood sugar.

8. Regular Meals:
- Consume regular meals and snacks to assist in keeping blood sugar levels steady. Blood sugar swings might result from missing meals.

9. Portion Control:
   - Be mindful of portion sizes to avoid overindulging, which may cause spikes in blood sugar.

10. Limit Processed Foods:
   - Minimize your consumption of processed and packaged foods, which often contain hidden sugars and unhealthy fats.

11. Monitor Blood Sugar:
   - Monitor your blood sugar levels as instructed by your healthcare provider to ensure they are within the target range.

12. Consult a Registered Dietitian:
   - Consult a qualified dietician with expertise in managing gestational diabetes. They can create a personalized meal plan and provide guidance on managing your condition.

13. Stay Active:
   - Incorporate regular physical activity, as advised by your healthcare provider, into your routine. Exercise can improve insulin sensitivity and assist lower blood sugar levels.

14. Gestational Diabetes Educator:
   - Consider attending sessions with a gestational diabetes educator who can provide comprehensive guidance on managing your condition.

15. Real Food Choices:
   - Focus on whole foods such as fresh fruits and vegetables, lean proteins, and unprocessed grains to create balanced, nutrient-rich meals.

Real food management of gestational diabetes emphasizes a balanced and nutrient-dense diet that minimizes blood sugar spikes and supports the health of both you and your baby. Be sure to consult with your healthcare provider and a registered dietitian for personalized advice and to monitor your progress throughout your pregnancy.

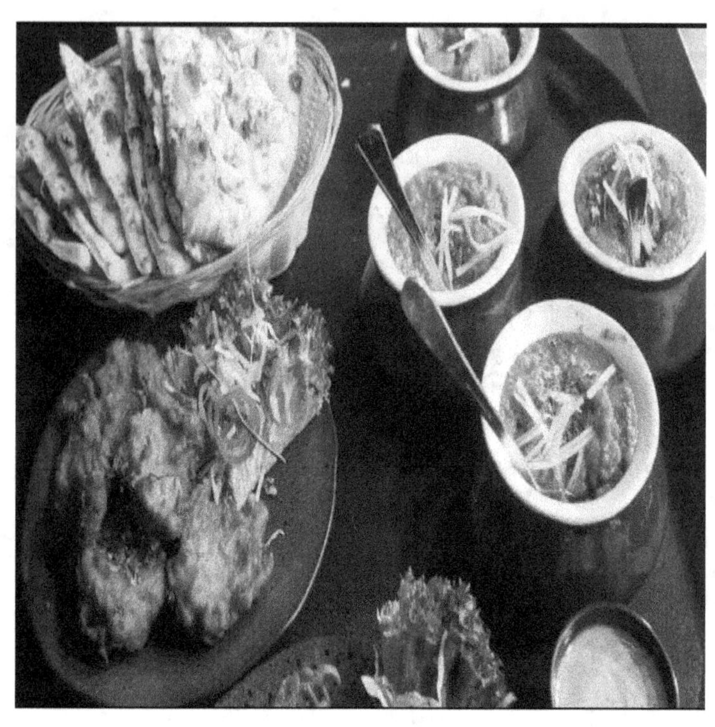

CHAPTER SEVEN

PREPARING FOR LABOR AND POSTPARTUM

Preparing for labor and the postpartum period is a crucial part of ensuring a healthy and comfortable pregnancy journey. Here are some essential considerations:

1. Childbirth Classes:
   - Consider enrolling in childbirth education classes. These classes can provide valuable information on labor, delivery, and postpartum care.

2. Birth Plan:
   - Draft a birth plan outlining your choices for the delivery, labor, and postpartum period. Discuss it with your healthcare provider to ensure alignment with your medical needs.

3. Choose a Healthcare Provider:
   - Select a healthcare provider (OB-GYN, midwife, or doula) who aligns with your birth plan and preferences.

4. Pack a Hospital Bag:
   - Prepare a hospital bag with essentials for labor and postpartum, including clothing, toiletries, and items for your baby.

5. Labor Support:
   - Decide who will be your labor support person, whether it's a partner, family member, or doula. Ensure they are well-prepared to assist you during labor.

6. Pain Management:
   - Discuss pain management options with your healthcare provider. These may include epidurals, natural pain relief techniques, or other methods.

7. Postpartum Support:
   - Plan for postpartum support, as you may need assistance with newborn care, household chores, and your own recovery.

8. Breastfeeding Education:
   - Consider taking breastfeeding classes to prepare for breastfeeding your baby. Knowledge and support can make a significant difference.

9. Infant Care Classes:
   - Enroll in classes or read up on infant care to become familiar with baby basics like diapering, feeding, and sleep routines.

10. Postpartum Care:
   - Understand what postpartum care involves, including the physical and emotional changes that occur after birth.

11. Mental Health:
   - Acknowledge the possibility of anxiety or postpartum depression. Reach out to your healthcare provider if you experience signs of these conditions.

12. Social Support:
   - Build a support network of friends and family who can provide assistance and emotional support during the postpartum period.

13. Postpartum Diet:
   - Consider postpartum nutrition to support your recovery and breastfeeding. Include nutrient-rich foods and stay well-hydrated.

14. Rest and Recovery:
   - Plan for adequate rest and recovery time after giving birth. This includes taking it easy and accepting help when needed.

15. Postpartum Fitness:
   - Consult with your healthcare provider about when it's safe to resume exercise and develop a postpartum fitness plan.

16. Babyproofing:
   - Begin babyproofing your home as your baby becomes more mobile.

17. Newborn Essentials:

- Ensure you have essential items for your baby, including a crib, car seat, baby clothes, and diapers.

18. Emotional Well-Being:
   - Focus on your emotional well-being during the postpartum period. Accept help, reach out for support, and prioritize self-care.

19. Birth Certificate and Legal Documents:
   - Ensure you have the necessary paperwork for your baby's birth certificate and any legal documentation.

20. Birth Announcements:
   - Plan how you want to announce the birth of your baby to friends and family.

21. Be Flexible:
   - Remember that birth and the postpartum period can be unpredictable. Be adaptable and willing to change your plans as needed.

Preparing for labor and the postpartum period is essential for a smooth transition into parenthood. Stay informed, communicate with your healthcare provider, and build a support network to ensure a positive experience during this transformative time.

REAL FOOD FOR LABOR

While it's important to stay nourished during labor, your body's needs are different during this intense and physically demanding process. Here are some real food options to consider:

1. Carbohydrate-Rich Snacks:
   - Simple carbohydrate-rich snacks can provide quick energy. Consider items like energy gels, honey sticks, or dried fruits.

2. Whole Grain Crackers:
   - Whole grain crackers can offer some sustenance without being heavy on your stomach.

3. Nuts and Seeds:
   - Nuts and seeds provide healthy fats and protein, offering longer-lasting energy. Almonds and chia seeds are good choices.

4. Fresh Fruit:
   - Slices of fresh fruit, like apple or watermelon, can provide hydration and a natural energy boost.

5. Protein Bars:
   - Choose protein bars with minimal ingredients and low added sugars to keep your energy up.

6. Hydration:

- Staying hydrated is essential. Drink water or electrolyte beverages to maintain your fluid balance.

7. Herbal Tea:
- Herbal teas like ginger or raspberry leaf tea can provide comfort and hydration.

It's important to consult with your healthcare provider and follow their recommendations during labor, as they may have specific guidelines for eating and drinking. Keep in mind that during active labor, your focus will be on the birthing process, and you may not feel like eating much. Choose light, easily digestible options that provide quick energy and hydration as needed.

POSTPARTUM NUTRITION AND RECOVERY

Postpartum nutrition and recovery are vital for replenishing your body's resources after giving birth. Here are some considerations for a healthy postpartum period:

1. Hydration:
- Stay well-hydrated, especially if you're breastfeeding. Drink plenty of water, herbal teas, and clear fluids to support milk production and recovery.

2. Balanced Diet:

- Aim for a balanced diet that includes a variety of nutrients. Consume fruits and vegetables, whole grains, lean meats, and healthy fats.

3. Nutrient-Rich Foods:
   - Choose nutrient-dense foods like leafy greens, nuts, seeds, and whole grains to support your recovery and overall health.

4. Iron-Rich Foods:
   - If you experienced blood loss during delivery, focus on iron-rich foods like lean meats, beans, and dark leafy greens to replenish your iron stores.

5. Omega-3 Fatty Acids:
   - Include foods high in omega-3 fatty acids, such as fatty fish (salmon, mackerel), flaxseeds, and chia seeds, to support your mood and overall well-being.

6. Fiber:
   - High-fiber foods can help prevent constipation, a common postpartum issue. Consume a lot of vegetables, fruits, and entire grains.

7. Protein:
   - Adequate protein intake supports healing and muscle recovery. Dairy products, legumes, and lean meats are excellent sources.

8. Snacking:

- Keep healthy snacks on hand for quick and easy access, especially if you're breastfeeding and need additional energy.

9. Vitamin and Mineral Supplements:
   - Continue taking any prescribed supplements, such as prenatal vitamins, if recommended by your healthcare provider.

10. Postpartum Depression:
   - Be mindful of your emotional well-being. Nutrient-rich foods and seeking support can help with mood stability.

11. Self-Care:
   - Prioritize self-care, which includes rest, relaxation, and adequate sleep. Ask for help from friends and family to manage household chores and childcare.

12. Slow and Gradual:
   - Allow yourself time for gradual weight loss and don't rush back into intense physical activity. Your body needs time to heal.

13. Breastfeeding:
   - If you're breastfeeding, be sure to nourish yourself properly, as your baby relies on your milk for nutrition.

14. Seek Support:

- Reach out for support from healthcare providers, lactation consultants, and mental health professionals if needed.

15. Mindful Eating:
   - Practice mindful eating, savoring your meals, and appreciating the nourishment they provide.

16. Nutrient-Dense Snacks:
   - Keep nutrient-dense snacks like yogurt, hummus, and cut-up vegetables handy for quick energy and nourishment.

17. Gradual Changes:
   - If you have specific dietary goals or changes you want to make postpartum, implement them gradually, considering your physical and emotional well-being.

Remember that the postpartum period is a time of significant adjustment. Prioritize self-care, rest, and proper nutrition to support your body's recovery and to provide the energy needed for caring for your new baby. Seek guidance from healthcare providers and consider working with a registered dietitian to create a personalized postpartum nutrition plan.

BREASTFEEDING AND BEYOND

Breastfeeding is a natural and beneficial way to nourish your baby, providing them with essential nutrients and promoting bonding. As you embark on this journey, consider the following tips:

1. Proper Latch:
   - Ensure your baby latches onto the breast correctly. Seek help from a lactation consultant if needed.

2. Frequent Feeding:
   - Feed your baby on demand, which may mean frequent nursing sessions, especially during the early weeks.

3. Stay Hydrated:
   - Drink plenty of water to maintain your milk supply and stay hydrated.

4. Balanced Diet:
   - Consume a well-balanced diet to support your own health and milk production. Nutrient-dense foods are key.

5. Rest and Recovery:
   - Prioritize rest and recovery. Breastfeeding can be physically demanding, and you need to care for your own well-being.

6. Breastfeeding Positions:
   - Explore different breastfeeding positions to find what's most comfortable for you and your baby.

7. Seek Support:

- Don't hesitate to ask for help and guidance from healthcare providers, lactation consultants, and breastfeeding support groups.

8. Pumping and Storing:
   - If you plan to pump and store breast milk, follow proper guidelines for storage and hygiene.

9. Weight Gain:
   - Keep track of your baby's weight gain to ensure they are getting enough milk.

10. Growth Spurts:
   - Be prepared for growth spurts, during which your baby may want to nurse more frequently.

11. Engorgement:
   - If you experience breast engorgement or discomfort, try warm compresses and gentle massage to ease the discomfort.

12. Sore Nipples:
   - If you have sore nipples, consider using lanolin cream or nipple shields to alleviate discomfort.

13. Weaning:
   - Decide when and how you want to begin weaning, as it can be a gradual process.

14. Beyond Breastfeeding:

- As your baby grows, introduce solid foods and wean from breastfeeding at a pace that suits you and your baby.

15. Emotional Support:
   - Remember that breastfeeding can be an emotional journey. Reach out for support if you experience difficulties or mood changes.

16. Birth Control:
   - Discuss birth control options with your healthcare provider while breastfeeding to ensure they are safe and compatible with your breastfeeding goals.

17. Breastfeeding Benefits:
   - Be aware of the many benefits of breastfeeding for both you and your baby, including bonding and immune system support.

18. Keep Learning:
   - Continue to educate yourself about breastfeeding to make informed decisions that align with your parenting style.

Breastfeeding is a unique and individual experience, and it's important to do what works best for you and your baby. Whether you breastfeed for a few months or for an extended period, it's a special bonding experience that provides invaluable nutrition and support to your baby's development.

CHAPTER EIGHT

THE REAL FOOD JOURNEY BEYOND PREGNANCY

The real food journey continues beyond pregnancy and into your postpartum and parenting years. Here's how you can maintain a commitment to healthy eating and a real food approach:

1. Family Meals:
   - Continue to prioritize family meals that focus on whole, unprocessed foods. These meals set a positive example for your children.

2. Meal Planning:
   - Plan your meals in advance to ensure that you consistently include real and nutrient-dense foods in your diet.

3. Teach Healthy Eating Habits:
   - Educate your children about the benefits of real food and help them develop healthy eating habits from a young age.

4. Avoid Processed Foods:

  - Reduce the amount of fast food and processed items you eat. Instead, prepare homemade, real food options for your family.

5. Cooking Together:
  - Let your kids help with food planning and cooking. This not only teaches them valuable skills but also encourages an appreciation for real food.

6. Balanced Diet:
  - Ensure that your family's diet remains balanced, incorporating a variety of fruits, vegetables, lean proteins, and whole grains.

7. Limit Sugars:
  - Be mindful of sugar intake and limit sugary snacks and beverages in your household.

8. Explore Local and Seasonal:
  - Support local and seasonal food sources whenever possible, as they often offer fresher and more nutrient-rich options.

9. Gardening:
  - Consider gardening as a family activity to grow your own fruits and vegetables, promoting a connection to the food you eat.

10. Food Education:
  - Continue to educate yourself about food and nutrition, staying updated on the latest research and guidelines.

11. Mealtime Habits:
   - Establish positive mealtime habits, such as eating together as a family and avoiding distractions like screens.

12. Snacking Choices:
   - Offer healthy snack options like fresh fruits, nuts, and yogurt to your children.

13. Real Food for Baby:
   - As your baby grows, introduce them to real food options, such as mashed fruits and vegetables, to encourage healthy eating habits.

14. Be a Role Model:
   - Set a positive example by following a real food approach yourself. Children are more likely to adopt healthy habits if they see you living them.

15. Family Involvement:
   - Involve your family in food decisions, such as planning meals and grocery shopping. Encourage open discussions about food choices.

16. Balance and Moderation:
   - Emphasize the importance of balance and moderation in eating. Teach your children to enjoy treats occasionally but prioritize nutritious foods.

17. Lifelong Learning:

- Encourage a lifelong love of learning about food, nutrition, and health within your family.

Your real food journey is not just about pregnancy; it's a lifelong commitment to healthy eating and well-being. By instilling real food values and habits in your family, you're setting the stage for a lifetime of good health and an appreciation for nutritious, whole foods.

RAISING A REAL FOOD FAMILY

Raising a real food family involves instilling healthy eating habits, a love for nutritious foods, and an appreciation for whole, unprocessed options. To help you with this, consider the following advice:

1. Start Early:
   - Begin teaching your children about real food from an early age. Introduce them to a variety of fruits, vegetables, and other whole foods as soon as they begin eating solids.

2. Be a Role Model:
   - Children learn by example. Be a positive role model by consistently choosing real food options and demonstrating a love for healthy eating.

3. Family Meals:
   - Make family meals a regular occurrence. Eating together promotes healthy eating habits and

provides an opportunity to connect with your children.

4. Involve Your Children:
   - Include your children in meal planning, grocery shopping, and cooking. This helps them feel connected to the food they eat and encourages them to make healthier choices.

5. Teach Food Education:
   - Educate your children about the benefits of real food and why it's important to choose nutritious options. Keep the information age-appropriate.

6. Limit Processed Foods:
   - Minimize the presence of processed and fast foods in your home. This makes healthy options the default choice.

7. Encourage Variety:
   - Offer a wide variety of fruits, vegetables, whole grains, and lean proteins. Try diverse dishes to add some excitement to your dinners.

8. Home Gardening:
   - Consider starting a family garden. Children often enjoy growing their own fruits and vegetables, fostering a connection to real food.

9. Snack Wisely:

- Keep nutritious snacks readily available, such as cut-up fruits and vegetables, yogurt, and nuts. Avoid stocking the pantry with unhealthy options.

10. Limit Sugary Beverages:
   - Encourage water and milk as primary beverage choices. Minimize sugary drinks, such as soda and excessive fruit juices.

11. Balance and Moderation:
   - Teach your children about balance and moderation in eating. Occasional treats are acceptable, but the focus should be on nutritious meals.

12. Avoid Food Shaming:
   - Refrain from criticizing particular dishes. Instead, emphasize the positive aspects of healthy choices.

13. Food Labels:
   - Educate your children about reading food labels to understand what's in the foods they eat.

14. Discuss the Origin:
   - Talk about where food comes from. This can help children develop an appreciation for the sources of their meals.

15. Encourage Questions:

- Encourage your children to ask questions about food and nutrition. Answer their inquiries honestly and with age-appropriate information.

16. Make Real Food Fun:
   - Experiment with fun and healthy recipes that involve your children, like making smoothies, homemade granola, or fruit kabobs.

17. Be Patient:
   - Be patient with picky eaters. It may take time for children to develop a taste for certain foods. Keep offering them without pressure.

18. Celebrate Food Together:
   - Create special occasions around food, such as picnics, family cooking nights, and trips to farmers' markets.

Raising a real food family is a gradual and ongoing process. By incorporating these strategies into your family life, you can instill healthy eating habits and a lifelong appreciation for nutritious, whole foods in your children.

SUSTAINABLE FOOD CHOICES

Making sustainable food choices is not only good for the environment but also supports your health and the well-being of future generations. Here are some strategies for choosing sustainably produced food:

1. Choose Locally Sourced Foods:
   - Opt for locally grown or produced foods. These products have a smaller carbon footprint because they travel shorter distances to reach your plate.

2. Seasonal Eating:
   - Prioritize seasonal fruits and vegetables. Eating in-season reduces the energy required for out-of-season produce.

3. Reduce Meat Consumption:
   - Reduce your consumption of meat and choose plant-based protein sources like legumes, nuts, and tofu. When you do eat meat, opt for sustainably raised and sourced options.

4. Sustainable Seafood:
   - If you eat seafood, choose sustainably sourced options that are harvested in an environmentally responsible manner. Seek certification labels such as the Marine Stewardship Council (MSC).

5. Organic and Non-GMO:
   - Support organic and non-genetically modified (GMO) foods when possible. These choices are better for the environment and can reduce the use of pesticides and synthetic fertilizers.

6. Reduce Food Waste:

- Plan your meals, use leftovers, and compost food scraps to reduce food waste.

7. Food Packaging:
   - Choose products with minimal and eco-friendly packaging to reduce plastic waste.

8. Support Sustainable Agriculture:
   - Purchase from farmers and companies committed to sustainable agricultural practices that prioritize soil health, crop rotation, and natural pest control.

9. Grow Your Own Food:
   - If you have space, consider starting a home garden to grow your own fruits and vegetables. It's a sustainable way to source fresh produce.

10. Avoid Overconsumption:
   - Practice mindful eating and avoid overconsumption. This reduces the demand for excessive food production and minimizes waste.

11. Eco-Friendly Cooking:
   - Use energy-efficient cooking methods and appliances to reduce your energy consumption in the kitchen.

12. Sustainable Food Choices for Children:
   - Teach your children about the importance of sustainable food choices from a young age,

fostering a lifelong commitment to eco-friendly eating.

13. Community Supported Agriculture (CSA):
   - Join a local CSA program to receive fresh, seasonal produce directly from local farms.

14. Support Sustainable Brands:
   - Choose brands and products that prioritize sustainability and ethical practices in their production and sourcing.

15. Food Certification Labels:
   - Look for certification labels like USDA Organic, Fair Trade, and Rainforest Alliance when shopping for food products.

16. Reduce Single-Use Plastics:
   - Avoid single-use plastic items like utensils, straws, and bags. Choose reusable and sustainable alternatives.

17. Educate Yourself:
   - Continue to educate yourself about sustainable food practices, as knowledge is key to making informed choices.

Making sustainable food choices is an ongoing journey. By incorporating these practices into your daily life, you can contribute to a more sustainable and environmentally friendly food system while also supporting your own health and well-being.

CONCLUSION

In conclusion, the journey of real food during pregnancy and beyond is an important and empowering one. By prioritizing whole, unprocessed foods, understanding your nutritional needs, and making sustainable food choices, you can not only support your own health but also contribute to the well-being of your baby and the environment.

Throughout this journey, remember the significance of balanced meals, mindful eating, and the importance of listening to your body. Embrace the joy of nourishing yourself and your family with wholesome, nutrient-dense foods.

As you navigate pregnancy, postpartum, and parenting, continue to educate yourself, seek support from healthcare providers, and inspire your family to embrace a lifestyle that values real food, nutrition, and sustainability. Your choices have a positive impact on both your immediate and future health.

Congratulations on your commitment to a real food approach, and may your journey be filled with health, happiness, and a love for delicious, nourishing meals.

EMPOWERING YOUR PREGNANCY JOURNEY WITH REAL FOOD

Empowering your pregnancy journey with real food is a wise and nurturing choice. By embracing whole, nutrient-dense foods, you're not only supporting your health and the health of your baby, but you're also making a positive impact on your overall well-being. It's crucial to remember the following:

1. Prioritize Nutrient-Dense Foods: Choose foods that are rich in essential nutrients, including fruits, vegetables, lean proteins, and whole grains. These provide the building blocks for a healthy pregnancy.

2. Balance Is Key: Strive for balanced meals that provide a combination of macronutrients (carbohydrates, proteins, fats) and micronutrients (vitamins and minerals). This balance is crucial for the well-being of both you and your baby.

3. Stay Hydrated: Proper hydration is essential during pregnancy. Drinking enough water is vital for various bodily functions and can help prevent common pregnancy discomforts like constipation.

4. Listen to Your Body: Pay attention to your body's signals and eat when you're hungry. Your appetite and nutritional needs may change throughout pregnancy.

5. Sustainable Choices: Make eco-conscious food choices by supporting sustainable and locally sourced options. The ecosystem and your health both gain from this.

6. Seek Professional Guidance: Consult with your healthcare provider and a registered dietitian to create a personalized nutrition plan that meets your unique needs during pregnancy.

7. Continue Postpartum: Your real food journey doesn't end with pregnancy. Continue making healthy, whole food choices as you navigate postpartum and parenthood.

Empowering your pregnancy journey with real food is a beautiful commitment to your health and the health of your baby. It's a step toward nourishing your body and creating a strong foundation for the future. Enjoy the journey and the delicious, wholesome meals that come with it.

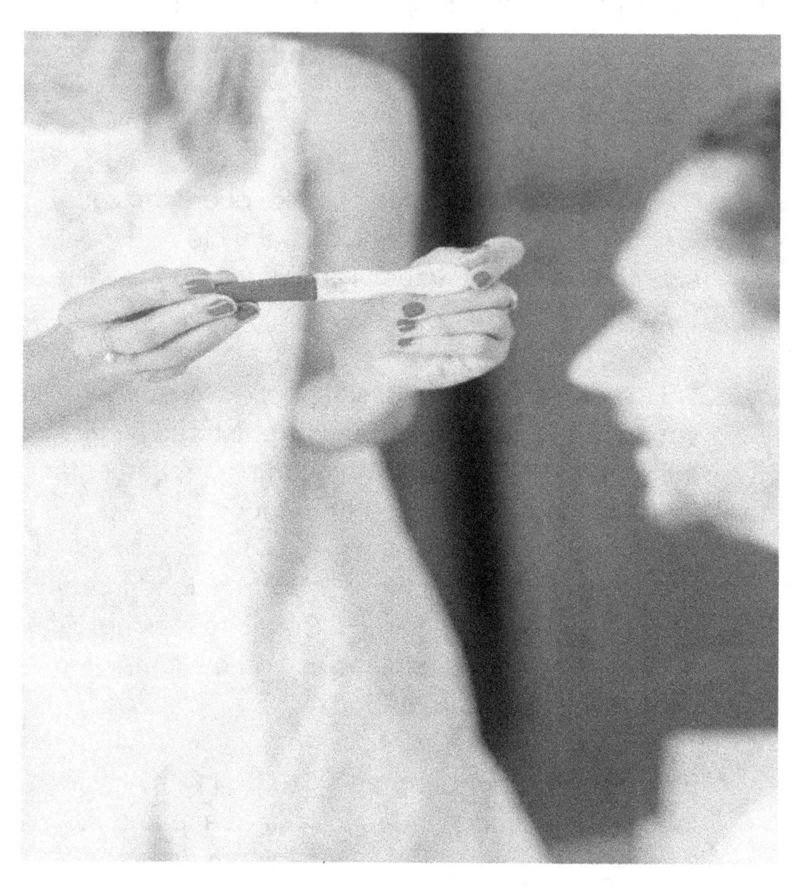